ALKALINE SMOOTHIE

Loose Stubborn Body Fat in 7 Days. Increase Energy, Boost Metabolism and Supercharge Your Health with Green Smoothie Recipes, Organic Smoothie, Detox Smoothie Recipes

Tamara White

ISBN: 9781731485519

TABLE OF CONTENTS

Mixed Berry Smoothie

Cacao Choco Cashew Milk

Creamy Hemp Milk

Chai Pumpkin Smoothie

Power Protein Smoothie

Carrot & Almond Protein Smoothie

Wicky Jelly" Smoothie

Quick Almond Butter Smoothie

Berry Lime Smoothie

Easy Weight Loss Smoothie

Energy-Booster Creamy Shake

Sunrise Smoothie

Blueberry Breakfast Smoothie

Alkaline Blended Smoothie

Alkaline Berries Morning Smoothie

Coarse Green Smoothie

Tahi Breakfast Smoothie

Chunky Green Smoothie

Alkaline Fat-Burning Smoothie

Creamy Chocolate PROTEIN SMOOTHIE

Friendly Green Smoothie

Green and Lean Protein Smoothie

Active Plain Smoothie

Cha Cha Smoothie

Dazzling smoothie

Strawberry Banana Moringa Smoothie

Banana Peach Sunrise Smoothie

Antioxidants Moringa Smoothie

Flavored Moringa Morning Smoothie

Moringa & Aloe Packed Smoothie

Camu Camu Berry Smoothie

Energy booster Protein Smoothie

Nutritious Hemp Berry Smoothie

Alkaline Chocolate Smoothie

Tropical Green Smoothie

Unique Detoxifying Green Smoothie

Healthy Workout Smoothie

Chocolate Mint Smoothie

Cranberry Breakfast Smoothie

Tangy Green Smoothie

Gorgeous Green Breakfast Smoothie

Glowing Alkaline Green Smoothie

Spinach, Mango Energizing Alkaline Smoothie

Justly Green Smoothie

Ginger Ale Green Smoothie

Alkaline Creamy Greens Smoothie

Quick Alkaline Creamy Greens

Lemon, Beet & Ginger

Refreshing Lime Lemon Shake

Mild Active Green Shake

Watermelon Strawberry Juice

Spackle Alkaline Smoothie

Banana and Apple Smoothie

Green Sublime Smoothie

Health Restoring Smoothie Recipe

Balancing Minerals Smoothie

Cally Smoothie

Multiple Function Alkaline Smoothie

Energized Wake-up Smoothie

Healthy Liver Revitalize Juice

Healthy Kidney Revitalize Juice

Almonds, Avocado Alkaline Smoothie

INTRODUCTION

What really is Alkaline Diet?

An alkaline diet — also called the alkaline acid diet, alkaline ash diet, acid alkaline diet, acid ash diet, and also called the pH diet — it assist in balancing the PH level of blood concerning the body fluids, including your urine and blood. Your pH is determined partially by the gravity of mineral properties of foods you eat. Every life forms and living organism rely on maintaining a proper pH levels, as the saying goes that there cannot be disorder and disease in a body with balanced PH.

The concept of acid ash assumption assist in making up the alkaline diet precept. Regarding research by Bone and Mineral expert, "The hypothesis of the acid-ash insinuates that grain and protein foods, having little potassium, generates a net acid excretion (NAE), let out calcium from the skeleton, generates more urine calcium, and diet acid load, which leads to osteoporosis.

The aim of the alkaline diet is the prevention of this kind of happening through consideration food pH levels, an effort to reduce dietary acid intake. Although this statement is not widely accepted by some experts, more than half all recognize that it is required by human life to have a tight regulated blood pH level of about 7.365 to 7.4.
Your pH can stay with the range of 7.35 to 7.45, it all depends on your diet, what you ate last, what time it is and time you went to the bathroom last.

WHAT IS AN ALKALINE SMOOTHIE?

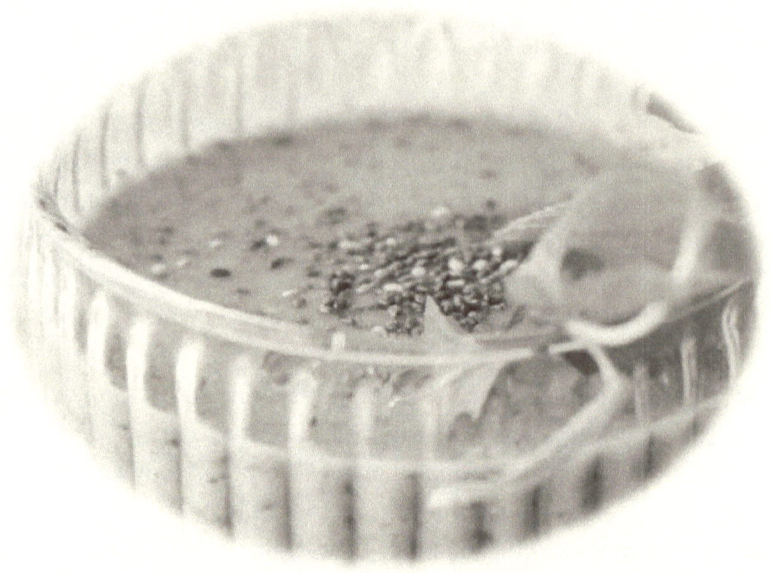

Alkaline smoothies are smoothie with high pH level, they are made from a blend of nutrient-rich ingredients like , kale, spinach, chai seed, avocado, leafy greens, bananas, berries and yogurt that are blended together to make a healthy alkaline forming smoothie. In general, it is best to use 40% greens and 60% ripe fruit, along few liquid to make blending easy.

Alkaline smoothies are fortified with good minerals and vitamins, they are loaded with satisfying fiber that can be changed for a meal and a huge volume of antioxidant.

Benefits of Introducing Alkaline Smoothie as part of your Diet

1. Keep out Unnecessary Ingredients

Making an alkaline ingredients does not need any cooking, with some few fruits and greens you have your healthy smoothie in no time.

2. Easy to Make

It's super easy to make an alkaline smoothie. It's simply done by combine your ingredients in a blender and in few minutes, you will be enjoying a pureed blend of nutrition.

3. Delicious Taste

That delicious smooth taste that comes from a combination of different healthy ingredients makes most people shocked about how lovely the taste is.

4. Easier to Digest

Blended makes the plant cells rupture, it becomes easily absorbed and digested by the body, which has nutritional benefit while supplying all necessary fiber needed to keep the system running with ease.

5. Keeps Your Body Alkaline

Alkaline smoothie helps to restore the pH level of yoyr body's to improve overall health. For best result, prepare your alkaline smoothie with alkaline water.

Alkaline water

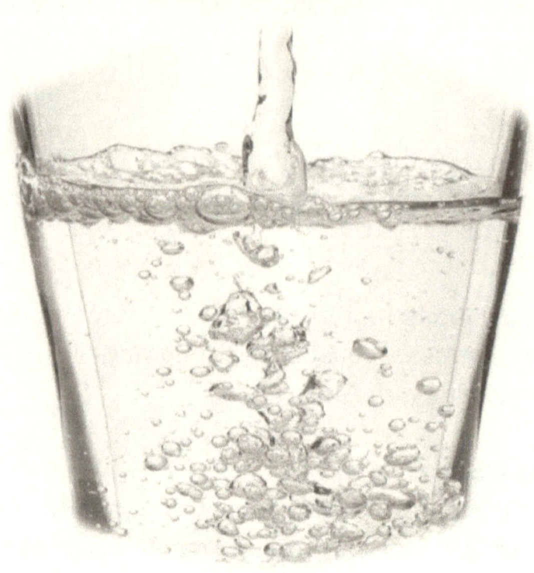

What is alkaline water?

What exactly do you understand by alkaline water? Some people believe it can help prevent chronic diseases, slow aging process, and regulate body's pH level.

Alkaline water is water that rich in alkalizing compounds, including bicarbonate, magnesium, potassium, silica, and calcium. Alkaline water has a higher pH level of 9 to 11 and also has less acidic than regular drinking water. It is believe that alkaline water can and help your body metabolize nutrients more effectively and also neutralize the acid in your bloodstream, leading to optimum health.

Benefits Of Alkaline Water

Helps prevent cancer
Weight loss
Detoxifying, skin health and hydration
Immune system support
Colon-cleansing properties
Anti-aging properties

What exactly is the meaning of "pH level"?

Potential of hydrogen (pH).This is a way of measuring acidity and alkalinity in the body. A measurement done on a scale of 0 to 14. If a solution is high in acidic, then the lower in PH. A higher alkaline, will result in a higher number. A PH of 7.4 is considered healthy, a PH of 7 is regarded as neutral, though PH levels are not all the same throughout the entire body, with the most acidic region being the stomach.

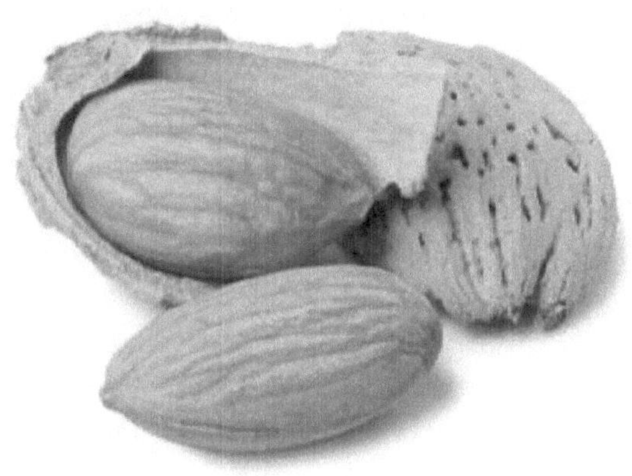

Any small alteration in the pH level of any organisms can pose a real challenge. For instance, as a result of increase deposition in the Carbon dioxide, the ocean' PH has reduced from 8.2 to 8.1 which is greatly affecting various ocean life forms. The pH level is very important to grow plants, hereby affecting the mineral composition of the foods we eat.

 Minerals in the human body, soil and ocean, are used as enhancer to maintain maximum pH levels, so a rise in acidity, results in a fall in minerals.

Testing Your PH for Alkaline Balance

Our major focus here is pH of your saliva, urine, and blood. Your blood must be tightly regulated at a constant pH of 7.365 and never changes.

Note: The purpose of this is not because you want to change your blood PH. When you test saliva or urine, the PH you get is for the fluid that your body eliminate and not the PH of your internal environment. It's needful that your body maintains a narrow range of PH of 7.365-7.45.Although there might be differences between the range you find in your saliva and urine as the body discharges plenty acids, which is a good thing for maintaining your internal PH. It might be more convenient to test your saliva than urine but urine reflects a better process of what the body undergo to eliminate acid from the body.

Saliva and Urine PH Testing

It's a very easy process testing your PH, at least it a good way to boost motivation and track your progress.
The saliva
Your saliva PH range is expected to be between 7.0 and 7.5
How to test Saliva PH:
Its best immediately you wake up in the morning before anything else or you can wait two hours after teeth brushing of food. Start by holding saliva in your mouth, swallow it and repeat a few times just to be certain your saliva is clean. Afterwards place some of the spit on a PH stip. A chart will be provided at the back of the kit, different shades of color reflects alkaline or acid state. Jot down the date, time and number to keep track of your progress.

How to test Urine PH

It shows the working performance of the body towards maintaining a proper PH blood. It reflects the body's effort, through the kidneys, lungs and adrenals in regulating PH by excretion of acids, and minerals like, sodium, calcium, potassium. Your urine PH range is expected to be between 6.5 and 7.5. A Ph of below 6.5 may indicate a system overwhelming.
This is also similar to the way you carry out your saliva test. Its best immediately you wake up in the morning you can urinate directly into a container and insert the PH strips or urinate on the Strip directly. A chart will be provided at the back of the kit, different shades of color reflects alkaline or acid state. Jot down the date, time and number to keep track of your progress.

How an Alkaline Diet works

Tips on how alkaline diets can be beneficial:
Because of the ratio of potassium to sodium in most people's diets which has dramatically changed, people consume now more sodium as potassium which are low in essential vitamins, antioxidants, fiber, magnesium and potassium. What most people consume now is simple sugars, refined fats, sodium and chloride. This has caused an increase in "metabolic acidosis" simply put, so many people PH level is low. The danger this pose is gradual loss of organ functions, it cause rapid aging, degenerates tissue, it cause the cells, bone, tissue and organs to loose important minerals.

Signs You've Got an Unhealthy Gut

Digestive discomfort, diahorrea, gas, and Bloating
Frequent feelings of anxiety
Inability to focus, lack of concentration and Poor memory
Depressive thoughts or ongoing depression
A short irritability/fuse and mood swings
Pre-diabetes or symptoms of Diabetes
Allergies
Already diagnosed autoimmune disease
Frequent use of antibiotics, or frequent infections
Topical skin complaints such as rosacea, eczema

List of Alkaline Smoothie Ingredients And Their Benefits

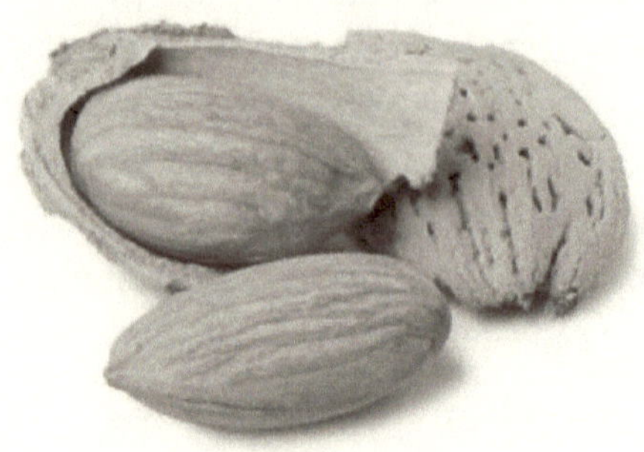

In order for the human body to function properly, it's necessary to maintain equilibrium, or homeostasis. To perform this, partly by maintaining pH, a way of measuring acidity and alkalinity in the body, also referred to as acid-base balance. To maintain the acid-base balance, what you eat plays a basic role. According to the research, a healthy diet is two-thirds base foods and one-third acid foods

Spinach

Fresh spinach: This powerhouse dark green veggie is loaded minerals benefits to the health. It is high in protein, fiber, zinc, iron, niacin and Vitamins K, E, C, B6, and A.

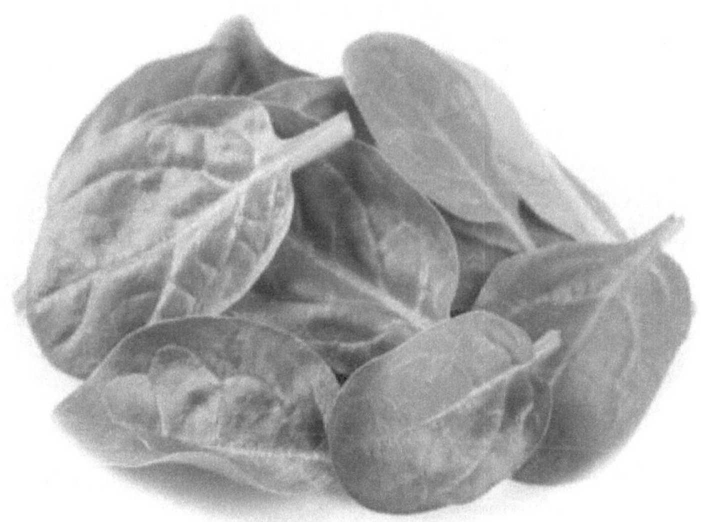

Kale: is very rich in alkaline-forming minerals, very beneficial to health. It is high in magnesium and calcium, also has high chlorophyll.

Berries

Berries, such as blueberries, blackberries, raspberries, and strawberries, are loaded with antioxidants and flavors. Though they have fructose, (a form of sugar) but also rich with minerals and vitamin. Fresh or frozen is good to use for your smoothies.

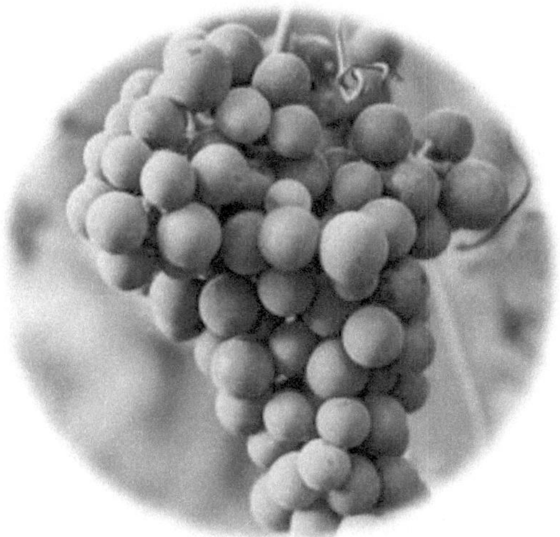

Banana

Bananas are amazing alkaline fruit to include in your smoothies. Ripe bananas have high alkaline level, don't hold back at using them. Bananas is also loaded with potassium.

Greek Yogurt

Yogurt contains healthy good bacteria like acidophilus, I rate this high as an alkaline-forming foods. Acidophilus helps to restores gut flora in the intestines. Yogurt aids easy food digestion. Unsweetened Plain Greek yogurt has no fruits added. It also gives a filling and creamy smoothies.

Dark, Leafy Greens like collard greens, turnip, romaine lettuce, kale, watercress and Swiss chard, and other dark, have high in folic acid (Folates). The rich vitamin-B prevent the cells from transform into cancer cells. Folates is good at preventing pancreatic and colorectal cancers.
Brussels sprouts and asparagus have good measure of folate.

Curcumin

This is ranked amongst the most potent cancer fighters. It decreases inflammation throughout the body and prevent against cancer. The ingredient contained in spice turmeric does double duty it makes it cancer cells very difficult for grow.

Garlic:

Garlic helps to reduce the risk of gastrointestinal cancers like stomach cancer, colon and esophageal.

Broccoli

This green super food is the highest in Sulphoraphane among cruciferous vegetables. That's the compound that flushes out cancer-causing chemicals and targets tumor growing cells.

Alkaline Diet Benefits

1. Protects Muscle Mass and Bone Density

Minerals is very important in maintaining and developing bone structure. The more alkalizing vegetables and fruits you eats, you stand a better chance at protecting yourself against muscle wasting as you age and decreasing bone strength "sarcopenia".
Following alkaline diet will help maintain minerals ratios crucial to maintaining lean muscle mass and build bones, including phosphate, magnesium and calcium, increase generation of vitamin D absorption and growth hormones, a way to protects bones and reduce plenty chronic diseases.

2. Help to Maintain a Healthy Weight
Increased eating of alkaline-forming foods and reducing the eating of acid-forming foods has been proven to prevent the body from obesity, it decrease inflammation and leptin levels, also affects fat-burning abilities and your hunger.

3. Protects Against Cancer and Helps Boost Immune Function
Lack of necessary minerals by the cells to fully oxygenate the body fully or dispose of waste, is dangerous to the body. Mineral loss will reduce vitamin absorption, pathogens and toxins will be accumulated in the body which damage the immune system.

4. Lowers Chronic Pain and Inflammation
Research has showed that there is a connection with alkaline diet and reduction in chronic pain.

5. Reduce Risk of Stroke and Hypertension
Alkaline diet performs an anti-aging effects on your body, is helps to push up growth of hormone production and decreases inflammation. It helps boost cardiovascular health and protect against issues like memory loss, stroke, kidney stones, hypertension and high cholesterol.

6. Kick against Magnesium Deficiency and Improve Vitamin Absorption
For the efficient functioning of volume of bodily processes and enzyme systems, an increase in magnesium is necessary. A lot of people are magnesium deficient, which can translate to anxiety, sleep troubles, headaches, muscle pains and heart complications. Presence of magnesium is needed to boost vitamin D and avert vitamin D shortage, essential to endocrine functioning and overall immune.

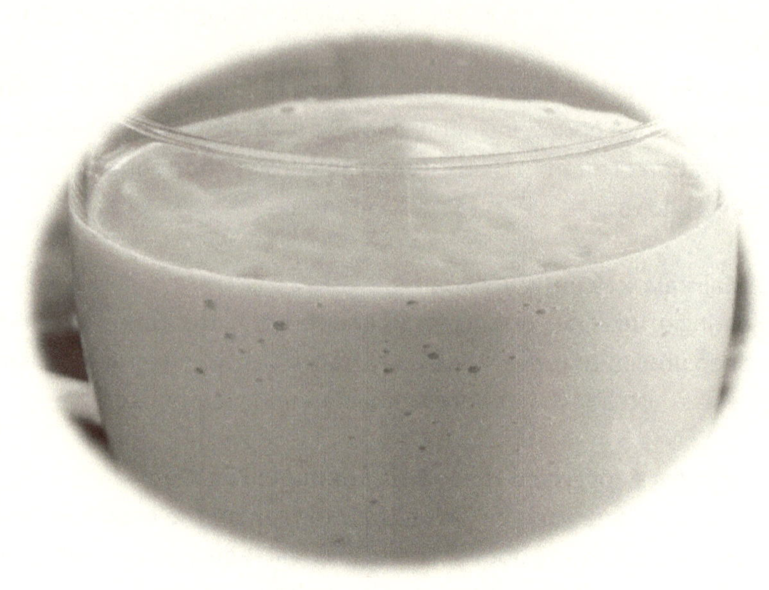

Some of the habits that can cause acidity in your body

Shallow breathing

Processed and refined foods

Poor eating and chewing habits

Pollution

Pesticides and herbicides

Over-exercise

Food coloring and preservatives

Chemicals Exposure and radiation from microwaves, cell phones, computers, building materials and household cleansers

Excess hormones from beauty products, foods, and health, and plastics

Excess non-grass-fed sources animal meats in the diet

Lack of exercise

Low levels of fiber in the diet

- Decreasing level of nutrient in foods because of industrial farming
- Chronic stress
- Artificial sweeteners
- Antibiotic overuse
- High caffeine intake
- Alcohol and drug use

ALKALINE SMOOTHIE RECIPES

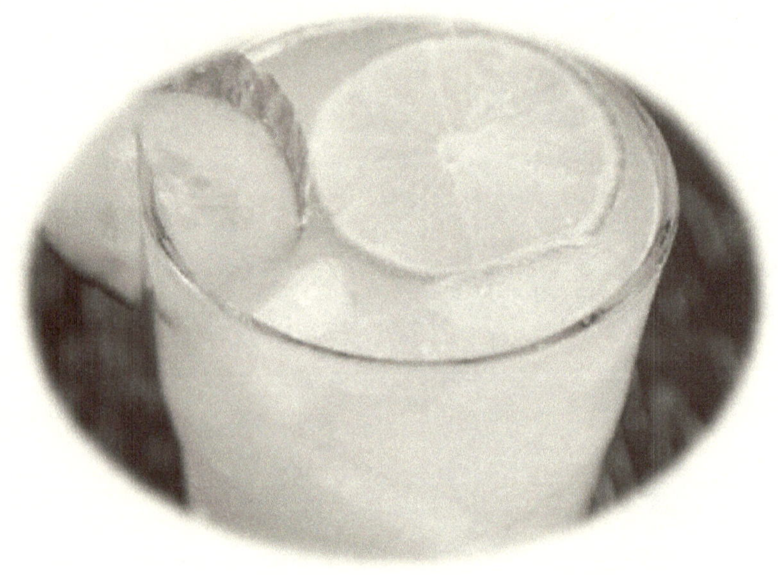

Jive Green Lentil Smoothie

Prep time: 5

Servings: 6

INGREDIENTS:

1/2 chopped cucumber

1 cup of chopped Kale, spines removed

3/4 cup red Lentils, cooked

1 medium cored and chopped Apple

1 medium Banana

1/2 cup chilled Water (preferably alkaline water)

3/4 cup Ice cubes crushed (preferably alkaline water)

1/2 cup of Greek yogurt, vanilla, fat-free

3 tablespoon of Honey

3 tablespoon of Lemon juice

1/2 tablespoon of Spirulina, dried

Preparations:

1. Combine all the ingredients in a blender blend until smooth.

Smooth Alkaline Super Green Shake

Serving: 1-2

INGREDIENTS:

Water (preferably alkaline water)

Cubes of ice, best made with alkaline water

1 tablespoon of SuperGreens Powder

1 peeled lime

1 cup of fresh spinach leaves

1 cup of cabbage

½ medium cucumber

1 avocado

Preparations:

1. With the exception of ice cubes and SuperGreens, combine all ingredients into blender, blend until smooth.

2 Serve on ice in a glass and add water as desired.

Cucumber Soy Shake with Coconut

Serving: 1
INGREDIENTS:
7 cubes of ice (best made with alkaline water)
1 teaspoon of organic vanilla
 2 small shredded cucumbers
50ml fresh unsweetened coconut milk, 500ml
Fresh unsweetened soy milk, 500ml
Preparations:
1. Combine all the ingredients in a blender blend until smooth in less 1 minute.

Green Power Cocktail

Serving: 2 shakes
INGREDIENTS:
½ cup of Wheat Grass
1 cup of Beets
1 cup of Kale
4 cups of Green Tops
4 cups of Sprouts
Preparations:
1. Use a juicer to extract all ingredients and enjoy cold or warm.

Alkaline Blackberry Smoothie

Serving: 2

INGREDIENTS:

½ teaspoon of vanilla

2 tablespoon of coconut oil

1 fresh lime juiced

1 large of bunch of kale

½ cup of frozen strawberries

1 cup of frozen blackberries

1 ½ cups of almond or coconut milk, unsweetened

1 tablespoon of raw almond butter (Optional)

Preparations:

1. Start by blending the coconut milk and kale first, then pour in the rest ingredients, and blend until you have a smooth mixture.

Seasonal Greens Smoothie

Prep time: 5 minutes

Serving: 1

INGREDIENTS:

1 tablespoon of coconut oil

Dash of cinnamon

1 chopped pear, preferably frozen

½ banana, preferably frozen

1 large handful of spinach

1 cup of coconut water

1 tablespoon of chia seeds (optional)

Preparations:

1. Combine all the ingredients in a blender blend until smooth

Mixed Cucumber Smoothie

Prep time: 5 mins

Servings: 2

INGREDIENTS:

1 cup Ice cubes, use alkaline water

1 1/2 cup of alkaline Water

3 drop of Stevia sweetener

2 tablespoon of fresh Lime juice

1/2 medium Jalapeno pepper (stemmed, seeded, de-ribbed)

1/8 Cucumber, peeled

1 medium stalk of Celery

Preparations:

1. Combine all the ingredients in a blender blend until you have a smooth mixture.

Fine Herbs With Green Smoothie

Prep time: 5 mins

Servings: 1

INGREDIENTS:

1/2 teaspoon of Chia seeds, ground (optional)

1 whole fresh Lime juice

1 cup of Water

1 1/2 tsp minced Ginger root (optional)

1/4 cup of diced Pineapple, banana or mango

1 medium Pear

2 medium Celery stalk

1/2 cup of Cucumber

1/2 cup of Cilantro (coriander)

1/2 cup of Kale

Preparations:

1. Combine all ingredients in a blender and blend until you have smooth mixture.

Green Biggie Smoothie

Prep time: 10

Servings: 1

INGREDIENTS:

1/4 cup of Water, alkaline

1 cup of Spinach

1 cup of diced Pineapple

1/2 cup of sliced Mango

1 cup of Kale, stems removed

1 cup of Ice cubes

1/2 Avocado

1 medium Apple

Preparations:

1. Combine all ingredients in a blender and blend, increasing the speed slowly until you have smooth mixture. Enjoy!

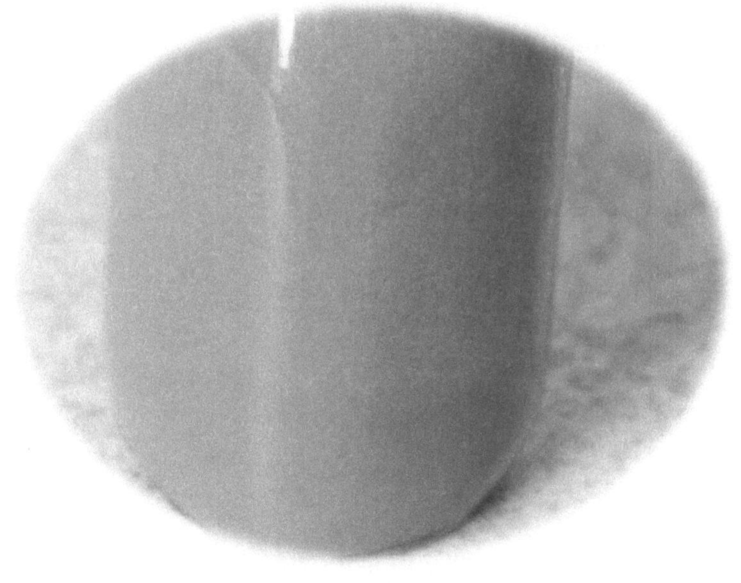

Mixed Berry Smoothie

Servings: 1

INGREDIENTS:

1 cup of coconut water

1 tablespoon of chia seeds

1 tablespoon of coconut oil

1 teaspoon of cinnamon

1 lime, freshly squeezed

1/2 frozen banana

½ cup of mixed frozen berries

1 large handful spinach

Preparations:

1. Combine all ingredients in a blender and blend until you have smooth mixture.

Cacao Choco Cashew Milk

Servings: 2

INGREDIENTS:

Optional: (80%) Cacao nibs or shaved cacao

Optional: 1 tablespoon of coconut butter

1 tablespoon of coconut oil

¼ cup of cacao powder

½ teaspoon of sea salt

1 teaspoon of cinnamon

1 teaspoon of vanilla

4 cups water

1 cup of cashews

Preparations:

1. Start by blending the cashews with 1 cup water for 30 seconds on high.

2. Add remaining 3 cups of water and the rest ingredients.

 Garnish with shaved cacao or cacao nibs. You can add ice to make it chill.

Creamy Hemp Milk

Servings: 2

INGREDIENTS:

Optional: 2 dates or/ and ½ banana and/or 1/4 cup raisins

Optional: ½ teaspoon of spice such as allspice, nutmeg, cardamom, or cinnamon

Optional: 2 tablespoon of cacao powder

Optional: Cheesecloth

⅛ Teaspoon of sea salt

½ tablespoon of coconut oil

½ teaspoon of vanilla extract

2 cups of filtered water

1 cup of shelled hemp seeds

Preparations:

Start by combining seeds and water, just enough to cover the seed, like an inch above into the blender.

2. Blend on multiple speeds to have a thick hemp cream.

3. Add the rest ingredients and blend again. 4. (Optional) Strain using the cheesecloth. Serve thick or add water in ratio 4.75 to 1 (water: hemp mixture).

Chai Pumpkin Smoothie

Servings: 2

INGREDIENTS:

1 tablespoon of chia seeds

1 date

1/4 teaspoon of nutmeg

1/4 teaspoon of minced or powder ginger root

1 teaspoon of cinnamon

1 frozen banana

1 cup of unsweetened pumpkin, canned or fresh (organic)

2 cup of unsweetened coconut or almond milk

2 cups of fresh spinach

Preparations:

1. Start by blending the almond milk and spinach first, with the exception of chia add rest ingredients and blend.

2. Add chia into the smooth mixture, then on a really low speed, blend to mix. Add chia and stir. Leave for a couple of minutes so the chia seeds can expand.

Power Protein Smoothie

Servings: 1

INGREDIENTS:

1 tbsp of hemp seeds

½ cup of blueberries (frozen)

1 tsp of cinnamon

Half banana

Organic Daily Protein Powder-Alkamind, 1 scoop

1 tbsp of almond butter

1 cup of unsweetened almond milk

Preparations:

Combine all the ingredients together in a Blender, blend until you have a smooth mixture. Enjoy your alkaline smooth

Carrot & Almond Protein Smoothie

Servings: 1

INGREDIENTS:

3 shredded carrots

1 tsp of cinnamon

Half banana

1 tbsp of almond butter

Organic Daily Protein Powder-Alkamind, 1 scoop

Half banana

1 tbsp of almond butter

1 cup of unsweetened almond milk

Preparations:

Combine all the ingredients together in a Blender, blend until you have a smooth mixture. Enjoy your alkaline smooth

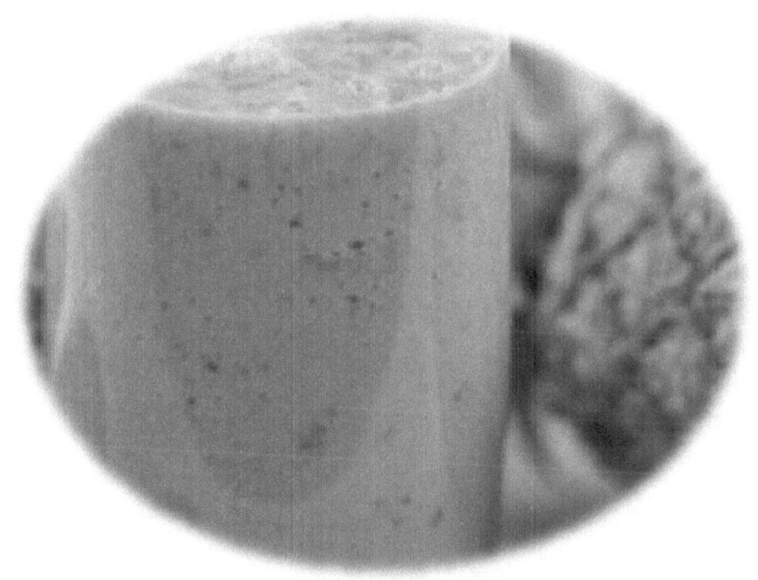

Wicky Jelly" Smoothie

Servings: 2

INGREDIENTS:

4 tablespoons of raw almond butter

1 banana, frozen

2 cups unsweetened almond milk

2 fresh cups of spinach

1 cup of mixed strawberries or berries (frozen)

Preparations:

Start by blending the almond milk and spinach first, then the rest ingredients.

Quick Almond Butter Smoothie

Servings: 2

INGREDIENTS:

1 tablespoon of chia seeds

4 tablespoons of raw almond butter

1 frozen banana

1 cup of frozen strawberries and frozen mixed berries

2 cups of unsweetened coconut or almond milk

2 cups of fresh spinach

Preparations:

Combine all the ingredients together in a Blender, blend until you have a smooth mixture. Enjoy your alkaline smooth

Berry Lime Smoothie

Servings: 1

INGREDIENTS:

1 tablespoons of chia seeds

1 cup coconut milk, unsweetened

1 scoop of Organic Daily Protein-Alkamind, Vanilla Coconut flavor (Optional)

2 tablespoons of fresh squeezed juice of lime

1 cup of frozen raspberries

1 handful of spinach

Preparations:

Combine all the ingredients together in a Blender, blend untill you have a smooth mixture. Enjoy your alkaline smooth

Easy Weight Loss Smoothie

Servings: 1

INGREDIENTS:

1 scoop of Organic Daily Protein-Alkamind (Creamy Chocolate)

1 cup of coconut or almond milk

1/4 teaspoon of sea salt (Himalayan, Redmond Real Salt or Celtic Grey)

1 teaspoon of fresh squeezed lemon juice

1/2 cup of frozen blueberries

1 frozen banana

1/4 cup of raw cacao powder

1/4 cup of golden flaxseed, ground

1/2 cup of raw almonds, soaked overnight

1 cup of spinach

Preparations:

Combine all the ingredients together in a Blender, blend until you have a smooth mixture. Enjoy your alkaline smooth

Energy-Booster Creamy Shake

Servings: 1

INGREDIENTS:

Half cup of ice

2 to 3 drops of organic stevia or 2 pitted dates

Optional: 2 teaspoons of maca powder

Quarter cup of raw cacao powder

Half haas avocado

1 tablespoon of raw almond butter

Half cup of almond milk, unsweetened

Preparations:

Combine all the ingredients together in a Blender, blend until you have a smooth mixture. Enjoy your alkaline smooth

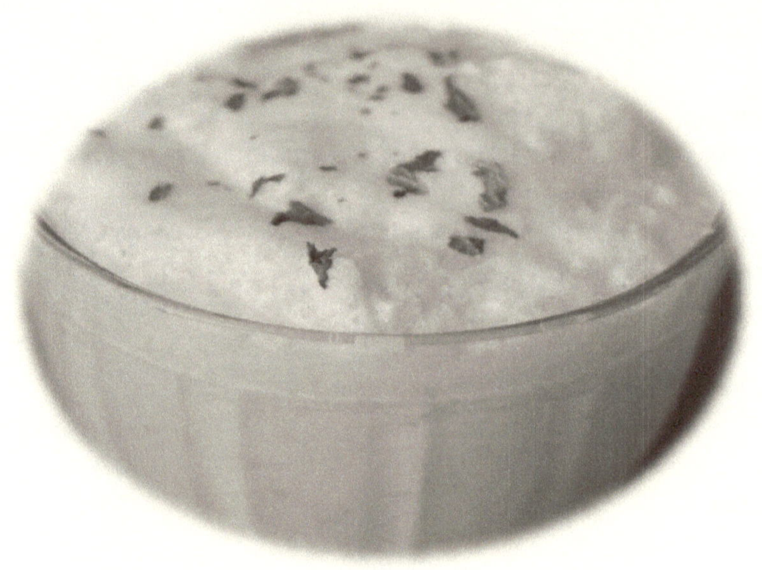

Sunrise Smoothie

Servings: 1

INGREDIENTS:

1 cup almond milk, unsweetened

1 tablespoon of coconut oil

1 tablespoon of flax or chia seeds

1 banana, frozen

½ cup of blueberries

2 cups of spinach

Preparations:

Combine all the ingredients together in a Blender, blend until you have a smooth mixture. Enjoy your alkaline smooth

Blueberry Breakfast Smoothie

Servings: 1

INGREDIENTS:

1 cup of coconut milk

1 tablespoon of coconut oil

1 tablespoon of hemp seed powder

1 tablespoon of ground flaxseed

1 tablespoon of chia

1 tablespoon of raw almond butter

½ cup of blueberries

1 handful of spinach

Preparations:

Combine all the ingredients together in a Blender, blend until you have a smooth mixture. Enjoy your alkaline smooth

Alkaline Blended Smoothie

Servings: 1

INGREDIENTS:

3 strawberries, frozen

1 ½ cups of coconut milk, unsweetened

1 tbsp of flax seeds

½ banana

1 cup of kale

¼ cup of basil

Preparations:

Combine all the ingredients together in a Blender, blend until you have a smooth mixture. Enjoy your alkaline smooth

Alkaline Berries Morning Smoothie

Servings: 2

INGREDIENTS:

¼ cup of fresh raspberries or frozen raspberries

1 cup of orange juice

½ cup of plain Greek yogurt

1 banana

½ cup of fresh strawberries or frozen strawberries

1 cup of kale

Preparations:

Combine all the ingredients together in a Blender, blend until you have a smooth mixture. Enjoy your alkaline smooth

Coarse Green Smoothie

Servings: 2

INGREDIENTS:

¼ cup of coconut water

½ cup of plain Greek yogurt

1 tbs of honey

2 tsp of shredded coconut

½ cup of mango

 ½ cup of pineapple

½ cup of spinach

Preparations:

Combine all the ingredients together in a Blender, blend until you have a smooth mixture. Enjoy your alkaline smooth

Tahi Breakfast Smoothie

Servings: 2

INGREDIENTS:

Ice (Optional)

1/2 cup of coconut water

1 peeled red grapefruit

1-inch crushed fresh ginger root

1/2 chopped cucumber

2 handful of spinach

1 avocado

Preparations:

Combine all the ingredients together in a Blender, blend until you have a smooth mixture. Enjoy your alkaline smooth

Chunky Green Smoothie

Servings: 2

INGREDIENTS:

Daily Greens, 1 Scoop

1 tablespoon of chia seeds

1/2 Cup of coconut water

1 chopped peach

1 Handful of spinach

1/2 Bunch kale

Ice (Optional)

Preparations:

Combine all the ingredients together in a Blender, blend until you have a smooth mixture. Enjoy your alkaline smooth

Alkaline Fat-Burning Smoothie

Servings: 2

INGREDIENTS:

Optional: 1 scoop of Organic Daily Protein-Alkamind (Vanilla Coconut flavor)

Some ice

1 tablespoon of chia seeds

1 tablespoon of raw almond butter

1 frozen banana

1 avocado

1 cup of unsweetened coconut milk or almond milk

Preparations:

Combine all the ingredients together in a Blender, blend until you have a smooth mixture. Enjoy your alkaline smooth

Creamy Chocolate PROTEIN SMOOTHIE

Servings: 1

INGREDIENTS:

1 cup almond milk or coconut milk, unsweetened

1 tablespoon of almond butter

1 medium beet

1 cucumber

1 scoop Daily Protein-Alkamind (creamy chocolate)

Preparations:

Fist shed the raw beet, then combine all the ingredients together in a Blender, blend and enjoy!

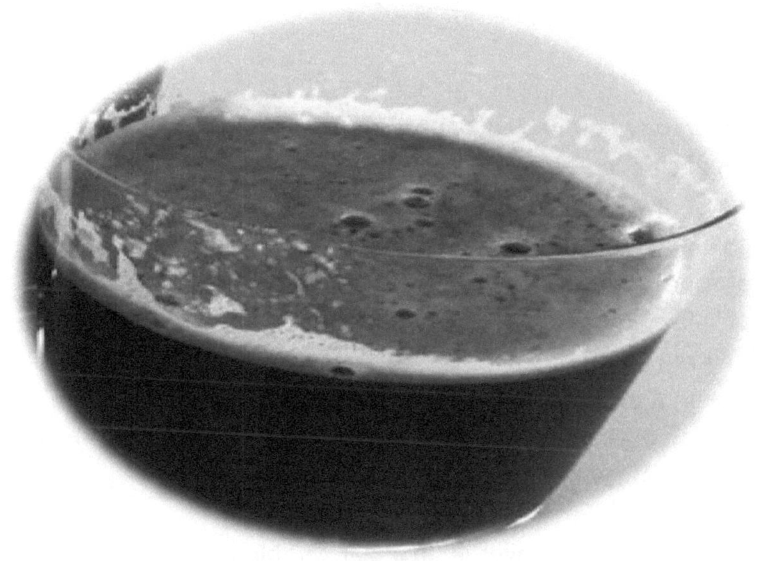

Friendly Green Smoothie

Servings: 1

INGREDIENTS:

Dash of cinnamon

4 drops of Vanilla extract

½ cup of almond milk, unsweetened

½ avocado

1 frozen banana

1 handful spinach

Preparations:

Combine all the ingredients together in a Blender, blend until you have a smooth mixture. Enjoy your alkaline smooth

Green and Lean Protein Smoothie

Servings: 1

INGREDIENTS:

1 tablespoon of unsweetened coconut flakes

1 tablespoon of chia seeds

1 tablespoon of raw almond butter

1 frozen banana

1 handful of spinach

1 handful of kale

3/4 cup of filtered coconut water

1/2 cup of coconut milk, hemp milk or almond milk

Optional: 1 scoop of Organic Daily Protein-Alkamind (Creamy Chocolate or Vanilla Coconut) you can sub with 1 tbsp. of hemp seeds, chia seeds, or/and flax seeds

Preparations:

Combine all the ingredients together in a Blender, blend until you have a smooth mixture. Enjoy your alkaline smooth

Active Plain Smoothie

Servings: 1

INGREDIENTS

Add 5 mint leaves (Optional)

1 tablespoon of hemp or chia seeds

2 tablespoon of raw cacao

2 tablespoon of raw almond butter

1/2 cup of ale

1 frozen banana

1 cup of coconut milk, hemp milk or almond milk

Preparations:

Combine all the ingredients together in a Blender, blend until you have a smooth mixture. Enjoy your alkaline smooth

Cha Cha Smoothie

Servings: 1

INGREDIENTS:

1 tablespoon of coconut oil

Optional: some Coconut ice

Optional: 1 frozen banana

1 cup of coconut water

4 ounces of fresh coconut meat

Preparations:

Blend all the ingredients together in a Blender and enjoy!

Dazzling smoothie

Servings: 1

INGREDIENTS:

1 cup raspberries, frozen

1/2 cup of frozen mango

1/2 cup of pineapple

1 cup of coconut water

Preparations:

Combine all the ingredients together in a Blender, blend until you have a smooth mixture. Enjoy your alkaline smooth

Strawberry Banana Moringa Smoothie

Servings: 1

INGREDIENTS:

Half or one tsp moringa leaf powder

2-3 dried dates or half tsp of maple syrup or honey

2 tbsp of vanilla Greek yogurt

One handful of strawberries

½ banana

1 cup of almond, coconut or soy milk, unsweetened

1 cup of raw spinach or kale

Preparations:

Combine all the ingredients together in a Blender, blend until you have a smooth mixture. Enjoy your alkaline smooth

Banana Peach Sunrise Smoothie

Servings: 1

INGREDIENTS:

1 tbs of moringa powder

1/2 cup of water

1/2 cup of coconut milk

1 tbsp of almond butter

2 bananas

1 cup of frozen peaches

Preparations:

Combine all the ingredients together in a Blender, blend until you have a smooth mixture. Enjoy your alkaline smooth

Antioxidants Moringa Smoothie

Servings: 1-2

INGREDIENTS:

1 cup of water

1 tsp of moringa powder

1 banana

½ cup of blueberries

½ cup of raspberry or strawberries

½ cup raw spinach

1/2 cup raw kale

Preparations:

Combine all the ingredients together in a Blender, blend until you have a smooth mixture. Enjoy your alkaline smooth

Flavored Moringa Morning Smoothie

Servings: 1-2

INGREDIENTS:

Some alkaline Water as desired

1 handful of raw oats

1/2 cup of Non-Dairy Milk

1 tbsp or less Moringa Powder

1-2 tbs of ground flaxseed

3-4 Fresh Pineapple Chunks

1 Banana

7-8 Blackberries, Frozen

Preparations:

Combine all the ingredients together in a Blender, blend until you have a smooth mixture. Enjoy your alkaline smooth

Moringa & Aloe Packed Smoothie

Servings: 1

INGREDIENTS:

1 tbsp of moringa powder

1 cup of aloe juice

1 cup of frozen or fresh pineapple

1 cup of spinach

Preparations:

Combine all the ingredients together in a Blender, blend until you have a smooth mixture. Enjoy your alkaline smoothie!

Camu Camu Berry Smoothie

Servings: 1

INGREDIENTS:

1 cup of Spinach (Optional)

1 teaspoon of camu camu powder

1 cup of almond milk

1 banana

2 cups of mixed berries, frozen

Preparations:

Combine all the ingredients together in a Blender, blend until you have a smooth mixture. Enjoy your alkaline smoothie!

Energy booster Protein Smoothie

Servings: 1

INGREDIENTS:

2 tbsp of hemp protein powder

¼ tsp of vanilla extract

1 tbsp of peanut or almond butter

1 cup of almond milk, unsweetened

1 large peeled banana

Preparations:

Combine all the ingredients together in a Blender, blend until you have a smooth mixture. Enjoy your alkaline smoothie!

Nutritious Hemp Berry Smoothie

Servings: 2

INGREDIENTS:

1 cup spinach

2 tbsp of hemp protein powder

1 cup of coconut milk

1 cup of mixed berries, frozen

1 large banana

Preparations:

Combine all the ingredients together in a Blender, blend until you have a smooth mixture. Enjoy your alkaline smoothie!

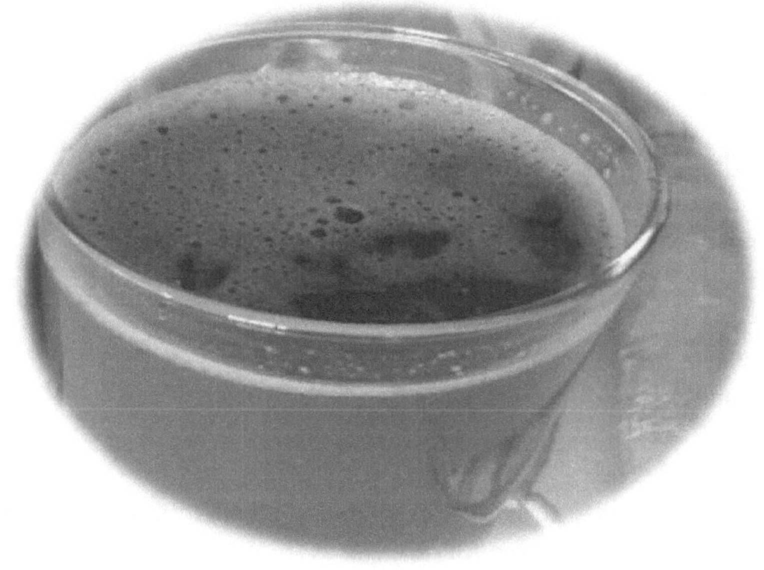

Alkaline Chocolate Smoothie

Servings: 1

INGREDIENTS:

1-2 tbsp of plain Hemp powder

1 cup of almond milk, unsweetened

1 tbsp of maple syrup (100% real)

3 tbsp of raw cacao powder (100% raw)

1 Avocado (peel and pitted)

1 cup of spinach

Preparations:

Combine all the ingredients together in a Blender, blend until you have a smooth mixture. Enjoy your alkaline smoothie!

Tropical Green Smoothie

Servings: 2

INGREDIENTS:

1 cup of coconut milk

1-2 tbsp of hemp powder

½ a lemon Juice

1 cup of papaya

1 cup of fresh or frozen mango

2 cups of spinach

1 avocado

Preparations:

Combine all the ingredients together in a Blender, blend until you have a smooth mixture. Enjoy your alkaline smoothie!

Unique Detoxifying Green Smoothie

Servings: 1

INGREDIENTS:

1 lime juice

1 cup ice

1 cup of coconut water

2 sprigs mint

1 cup of chopped cucumber

1 fresh or frozen mango

1 handful of spinach

Preparations:

Combine all the ingredients together in a Blender, blend until you have a smooth mixture. Enjoy your alkaline smoothie!

Healthy Workout Smoothie

Servings: 1

INGREDIENTS:

¼ cup of almonds

1 ½ cups of coconut water

1 inch ginger

1 tbsp of hemp seeds

½ cup of fresh or frozen Mango

1 cup of Kale

Preparations:

Combine all the ingredients together in a Blender, blend until you have a smooth mixture. Enjoy your alkaline smoothie!

Chocolate Mint Smoothie

Servings: 2

INGREDIENTS:

1 cup of coconut ice

1 teaspoon of chia

½ small avocado

½ cup of packed mint leaves

(Optional) 2 tablespoon of cacao nibs

1/4 cup of raw cacao

1 cup of almond or coconut milk, (or more)

4 dates pitted

¼ cup of soaked raw almonds (best to soak overnight)

Preparations:

Combine all the ingredients with the exception of chia together in a Blender, blend until you have a smooth mixture. Add chai, mix and enjoy your alkaline smoothie!

Cranberry Breakfast Smoothie

Servings: 2

INGREDIENTS:

½ cup of ice cubes

1 date, pitted

1/8 teaspoon of cinnamon

2 teaspoon of grated ginger or 1 inch piece of ginger root

2 tablespoons of fresh lemon juice

1 haas avocado

1 cup of fresh spinach

1 cup of organic or frozen cranberries

½ cup of soaked raw almonds (best to soak overnight)

2 cups of coconut water

Preparations:

Combine soaked almond, spinach and a little water in a Blender, blend to smooth. Add the rest ingredient and blend until you have a smooth mixture. Enjoy your alkaline smoothie!

Tangy Green Smoothie

Servings: 1

INGREDIENTS:

2 green apple slices

¼ juice of lime

¼ juice of lemon

1 inch of ginger

1 handful of parsley

1 stalk of celery

¼ cucumber

½ bunch of kale

1 handful of spinach

Preparations:

Combine all the ingredients together in a Blender, blend until you have a smooth mixture. Enjoy your alkaline smoothie!

Gorgeous Green Breakfast Smoothie

Servings: 1

INGREDIENTS:

1 tablespoon of chia seeds

½ cup of coconut water

½ cup of peaches

½ cup of strawberries

½ cucumber

1 handful of spinach

½ bunch of kale

Preparations:

Combine all the ingredients together in a Blender, blend until you have a smooth mixture. Enjoy your alkaline smoothie!

Glowing Alkaline Green Smoothie

Servings 2 16-ounce glasses

INGREDIENTS:

2 cups ice cubes

Pinch of sea salt

20 drops of liquid stevia (alcohol-free) plus more to taste

2 peeled medium limes, halved

1 tsp of lime zest, finely grated

1/2 roughly chopped English cucumber

1 peeled and pitted medium avocado

1 cup (180g) young Thai coconut meat

2 (88g) cups of tightly packed baby spinach

3/4 (180ml) cup of filtered water or raw coconut water

Optional boosters:

1/2 tsp of probiotic powder

1 tsp of wheatgrass powder

1 tbsp of virgin coconut oil

1/4 cup of raw broccoli florets (frozen)

Preparations:

Combine all the ingredients together in a Blender, blend on high for 30 to 60 seconds until you have a smooth mixture. Tweak stevia to taste. Enjoy your alkaline smoothie!

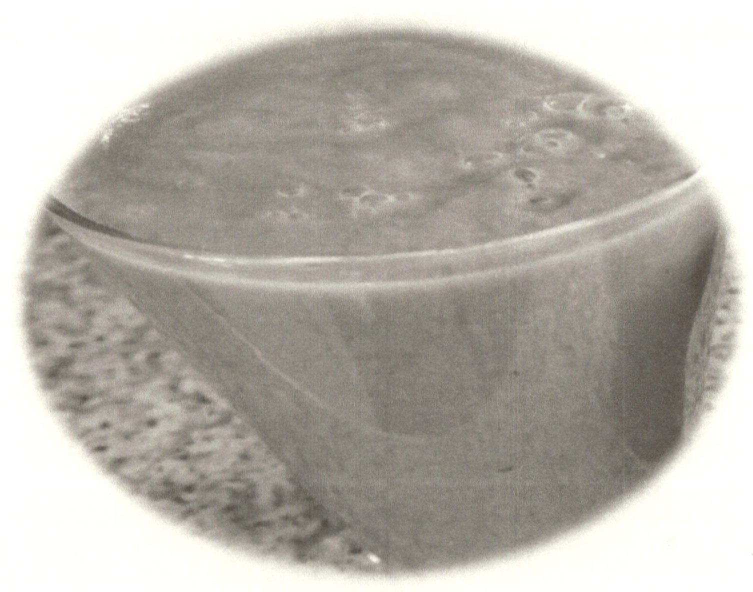

Spinach, Mango Energizing Alkaline Smoothie

Servings: 1

INGREDIENTS:

1 cup of water

1 juice of lemon, leave pith on

2 ginger (thumb sized knobs)

1/2 cup of chopped mango, frozen

1 banana

1 handful of spinach

2 large Tuscan kale leaves

Preparations:

Combine all the ingredients together in a Blender, blend until you have a smooth mixture. Enjoy your alkaline smoothie!

Justly Green Smoothie

Servings: 1

INGREDIENTS:

Few bok Choy stems

1 stalk celery

1 peeled lemon

1 fennel piece

1 cucumber

Preparations:

Combine all the ingredients together in a Blender, blend until you have a smooth mixture. Enjoy your alkaline smoothie!

Ginger Ale Green Smoothie

Servings: 1

INGREDIENTS:

1 peeled lemon

1/2 in piece of ginger

2 kale leaves

Few parsley stem

Few mint stems

1 cucumber

Preparations:

Combine all the ingredients together in a Blender, blend until you have a smooth mixture. Enjoy your alkaline smoothie!

Alkaline Creamy Greens Smoothie

Servings: 1-2

INGREDIENTS:

1-2 tsp of Bragg's soy sauce

Pinch of sea salt

1 small clove garlic

1 avocado

Few parsley stems & basil stems

1 small cabbage wedge

3-4 inches parsnip piece

Few bok choy stems

1 celery stalk

Few stems of broccoli

1 cucumber

Preparations:

1. Start by combining cucumber, parsley, basil, cabbage, parsnip, choy and broccoli into the blender, blend until smooth the add 1-2 tsp of Braggs soy sauce, pinch of sea salt, 1 small clove garlic, and 1 avocado. Blend until you have a smooth mixture. Enjoy your alkaline smoothie.

Quick Alkaline Creamy Greens

Servings: 1

INGREDIENTS:

Few parsley stems & basil stems

1 small cabbage wedge

3-4 inches parsnip piece

Few bok choy stems

1 celery stalk

Few stems of broccoli

1 cucumber

Preparations:

Combine all the ingredients together in a Blender, blend until you have a smooth mixture. Enjoy your alkaline smoothie!

Lemon, Beet & Ginger

Servings: 1

INGREDIENTS:

1 1/2 inch of ginger

1 peeled lemon

4 medium peeled beets

Preparations:

Combine all the ingredients together in a Blender, blend until you have a smooth mixture. Enjoy your alkaline smoothie!

Refreshing Lime Lemon Shake

Servings: 3

INGREDIENTS:

Pinch of sea salt

¼ cup lime juice

½ cup lemon juice

¼ ounces of Stevia powder

4 cup of young Thai coconut water

1 ½ cup of roughly chopped young Thai coconut meat

1 large roughly chopped cucumber

1½ roughly chopped Hass avocado

Preparations:

Combine all the ingredients together in a Blender, blend until you have a smooth mixture. Enjoy your alkaline smoothie!

Mild Active Green Shake

Servings: 2

INGREDIENTS:

½ large cucumber

1 ounce of lime juice

6 ounces of grapefruit juice

1 Hass avocado

½ lb spinach

4 ounces of raw coconut milk

1 teaspoon of Super Greens Powder

1 teaspoon of soy sprout powder or hemp protein powder

10 drops prime pH Drops

4 sprigs of fresh mint

14 cubes purified water ice

Preparations:

Combine all the ingredients together in a Blender, blend until you have a smooth mixture. Enjoy your alkaline smoothie!

Watermelon Strawberry Juice

Servings: 3

INGREDIENTS:

2 cups of Strawberries frozen

1 Lemon Juice

2 Cups of Watermelon

Preparations:

Combine all the ingredients together in a Blender, blend until you have a smooth mixture. If you prefer your juice not having pulp, you can also strain using a nut milk bag. Enjoy your alkaline smoothie!

Spackle Alkaline Smoothie

Servings: 2

INGREDIENTS:

1 cup of ice

1 tsp of chia seeds

1 handful of spinach fresh

5 frozen strawberries

1/2 small banana

1 cup of cubed watermelon

1 cup of almond milk

Preparations:

1. Combine spinach, chai seed banana and 1/2 almond milk and ice in a blender. Blend until smooth.

2. Then blend the almond milk, ice, watermelon, and strawberries together.

3. Combine the smoothies together in a glass and enjoy.

Banana and Apple Smoothie

Servings: 1

INGREDIENTS:

1 tsp of vanilla extract
1/2 cup of ice
1 1/2 tbsp of hemp seeds
1/2 tsp of cinnamon
1 small frozen banana
1 small apple
1 cup of almond milk

Preparations:

Combine all the ingredients together in a Blender, blend until you have a smooth mixture. Top with additional hemp seeds if you wish. Enjoy your alkaline smoothie!

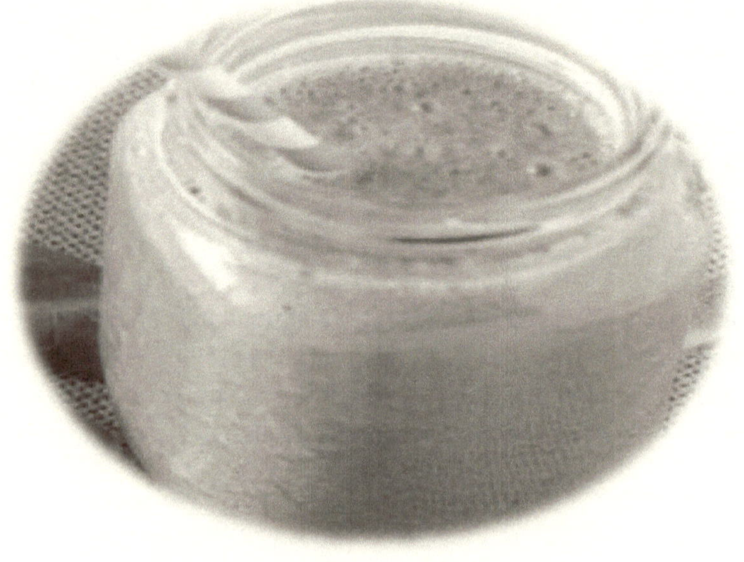

Green Sublime Smoothie

Servings: 1

INGREDIENTS

1 Lemon (I prefer Meyer)

¾ Cups Cold water

4 Stalks of Celery

1 Green apple

1 Pear

1 Ripe banana

1 romaine lettuce Head

1 Bunch of Baby spinach

Preparations:

Combine all the ingredients together in a Blender, blend until you have a smooth mixture. Enjoy your alkaline smoothie!

Health Restoring Smoothie Recipe

Servings: 2

INGREDIENTS:

2 tablespoon of chia seeds

Half cup of almonds (best to soak overnight)

Half cucumber

1 handful of spinach

100ml of filtered water

200ml of dairy replacement version coconut milk (from a carton) – not the thick canned version

1/4 teaspoon of dried TUNERIC or 1/2 inch of fresh turmeric

Half bunch OF parsley

1 dessert spoon OF coconut oil

1 avocado

Preparations:

Combine all the ingredients together in a Blender, blend until you have a smooth mixture. Enjoy your alkaline smoothie!

Balancing Minerals Smoothie

Servings: 2

INGREDIENTS

Pinch of Himalayan pink salt

1 tablespoon of coconut oil

1/8 teaspoon of ground cardamom

1/8 teaspoon of ground nutmeg

1/4 teaspoon of ground ginger

1/2 teaspoon of ground Ceylon cinnamon

1 tablespoon of cashew butter

Half avocado

1 tablespoon of chia seeds

Handful of almonds, (best soaked overnight and rinse)

150ml of filtered water

350ml coconut or almond milk, unsweetened

1 scoop of plant based protein powder (Optional)

Preparations:

Combine the soaked almonds, almond or coconut milk and water in the blender and blend until you have a smooth mixture, then add the rest ingredients. Enjoy your alkaline smoothie!

Cally Smoothie

Servings: 1

INGREDIENTS:

Coconut or Filtered Water

250ml Coconut or Almond Milk

Handful Swiss chard

Handful of Spinach

1 Cucumber

1 tablespoon of Almonds

1 tablespoon of Sesame Seeds

1 tablespoon of Pumpkin Seeds

Handful Kale

1/2 Avocado

INGREDIENTS:

Combine all the ingredients together in a Blender add the Coconut or filtered Water towards the end to get to the consistency you desire.

Multiple Function Alkaline Smoothie

Servings 2

INGREDIENTS:

2 carrots

Filtered water

1 small beetroot

1 red capsicum

1 teaspoon of powdered or 2 cm turmeric

1 inch or less ginger

2 sticks of celery

Half cucumber slice

2 handfuls of kale

4 handfuls of spinach

 4 handfuls of spinach

Preparations:

Combine all the ingredients together in a Blender add the Coconut or filtered water towards the end to get to the consistency you desire.

Energized Wake-up Smoothie

Servings: 2

INGREDIENTS:

200ml of almond milk

1/2 cup of navy beans

Handful of pumpkin seeds

(approx. 25 nuts) Small handful of almonds

3 handfuls of Swiss chard

4 handfuls of spinach

1 small cucumber

3 handfuls of kale

1 avocado

 1/2 Inch Ginger

Preparations:

Combine all the ingredients together in a Blender, blend until you have a smooth mixture. Enjoy your alkaline smoothie!

Healthy Liver Revitalize Juice

Servings: 2

INGREDIENTS:

1 Carrot

1 Beetroot

1 Inch Turmeric

1/2 Inch Ginger

1/2 Grapefruit

2 Handfuls of Spinach

1/2 Bunch of Kale

1 Cucumber

Preparations:

1. Start by juicing, the spinach, the turmeric and ginger, then the root vegetables, and cucumber lastly. Add the Coconut or filtered water towards the end to wash everything down.

2. Lastly, squeeze and mix in the grapefruit gently.

Healthy Kidney Revitalize Juice

Serving: 2

INGREDIENTS:

200ml coconut of water

1 cucumber

2 handfuls of kale

1 red capsicum

1cm of ginger root

1cm of turmeric root

Preparations:

Combine all the ingredients together in a Blender, blend until you have a smooth mixture. Enjoy your alkaline smoothie!

Almonds, Avocado Alkaline Smoothie

Servings: 2

INGREDIENTS:

200ml filtered water

200ml of unsweetened almond milk

1 teaspoon of almond butter

1 tablespoon of chia seeds

1 tablespoon of coconut oil

1/2 Cup of almonds (best to soak overnight)

2 Handfuls of kale

2 Handfuls of baby spinach leaves

1/2 Avocado

Preparations:

Combine all the ingredients together in a Blender with the exception of chai, blend until you have a smooth mixture. Stir in the chai and then wait for 2 minutes. Enjoy your alkaline smoothie!